Night Time Yoga
For
working Women

Deep Relaxation: Yoga Nitra:
Self-Care Ritual :gentle Stretches

By
Ellie Grace

Table of Contents

Introduction

In the clamoring beat of current life, working ladies frequently end up shuffling numerous obligations, from proficient responsibilities to family obligations and individual goals. In the midst of this hurricane, it's not difficult to disregard taking care of oneself and focus on all the other things over our own prosperity. Be that as it may, taking care of oneself isn't simply an extravagance; it's a need, particularly for ladies who are continually exploring through the requests of day to day existence.

Yoga, an old practice that fits the body, psyche, and soul, offers a safe-haven of serenity in the midst of the tumult. While yoga is helpful whenever of the day, rehearsing it at night or before sleep time holds specific importance for working ladies. Evening time yoga fills in as a scaffold between the requests of the day and the peacefulness of the evening, assisting ladies with loosening up, discharge pressure, and get ready both intellectually and truly for helpful rest.

In this aide, we will investigate the significant advantages of integrating evening time yoga into the existences of working ladies. From easing pressure and facilitating muscle strain to advancing unwinding and upgrading rest quality, evening yoga offers a heap of benefits that resound profoundly with the special difficulties looked by ladies in the labor force.

As we dive further into the act of evening yoga, we will reveal an assortment of delicate yet strong yoga successions explicitly customized to address the requirements of working ladies. These groupings will zero in on delivering developed pressure in key region of the body, quieting the psyche, and sustaining a feeling of internal harmony and equilibrium. Whether you're a carefully prepared yogi or a novice to the training, these groupings are intended to be open and versatile to ladies of all degrees of involvement and wellness.

Moreover, we will investigate the significance of developing a careful sleep time schedule that goes past yoga alone. From integrating unwinding procedures, for example, profound breathing and reflection to establishing a mitigating climate helpful for rest, we will reveal techniques to assist working ladies with embracing the change from the heftiness of the day to the peacefulness of the evening.

Additionally, we will inspect the science behind the significant effect of evening yoga on both physical and mental prosperity. From its capacity to direct the autonomic sensory system and lessen cortisol levels to its part in advancing the development of rest actuating chemicals like melatonin, the remedial impacts of evening time yoga are grounded in logical proof.

At last, this guide means to enable working ladies to focus on their taking care of oneself and recover their nights as a holy time for revival and recharging. By embracing the act of evening time yoga, ladies can develop a more profound association with themselves, sustain their bodies and psyches, and explore the intricacies of present day existence with beauty and flexibility. As we set out on this excursion together, may we track down comfort in the delicate hug of the evening and stir to a more splendid, more dynamic variant of ourselves every morning.

Chapter no 1
Unwind With Evening Stretches

In the present quick moving world, it's not difficult to wind up wrecked by the requests of day to day existence. From work cutoff times to family obligations, the buzzing about can negatively affect our bodies and brains. Be that as it may, in the midst of the turmoil, focusing on taking care of oneself and relaxation is essential. One successful method for loosening up and restore is through night extends. These delicate activities not just assistance to deliver pressure amassed over the course of the day yet additionally advance adaptability, versatility, and generally prosperity. In this aide, we'll investigate the advantages of night extends and give a thorough daily practice to help you loosen up and feel revived.

The Advantages of Night Stretches:

Stress Alleviation:
Evening stretches can assist with lightening pressure by advancing unwinding and diminishing muscle strain. As you stretch your muscles, you discharge developed pressure and strain, permitting you to feel more quiet.
Further developed Adaptability: Normal extending can further develop adaptability by expanding the scope of movement in your joints. This can assist with forestalling wounds and work on generally speaking portability.

Better Rest:
Participating in delicate extending before bed can assist with advancing better rest quality. Extending assists

with loosening up both the body and brain, making it more straightforward to nod off and stay unconscious over the course of the evening.

Decreased Muscle Touchiness:

On the off chance that you've had a drawn out day or taken part in actual work, extending can assist with mitigating muscle touchiness and firmness. By delicately extending tight muscles, you advance blood stream and course, which helps with recuperation.

Upgraded Brain Body Association:

Extending isn't only valuable for the body; it additionally advances care and attention to the current second. As you center around your breath and the impression of extending, you develop a more profound association between your body and brain.

Evening Stretches Schedule:

Prior to starting any extending schedule, it's fundamental for warm up your muscles with some light action, like strolling or delicate developments. Whenever you're heated up, find a tranquil, agreeable space where you can extend without interruptions. Make sure to inhale profoundly and carefully all through the stretches, and never drive yourself into torment. Pay attention to your body and change the stretches on a case by case basis.

Neck Stretch:

Sit or stand tall with your shoulders loose.

Delicately slant your head aside, bringing your ear towards your shoulder.

Hold for 15-30 seconds, feeling a delicate stretch at the edge of your neck.

Rehash on the opposite side.

Shoulder Stretch:

Broaden one arm across your body at shoulder level.

Utilize your other hand to press the arm towards your chest, feeling a stretch in the shoulder and upper back delicately.

Hold for 15-30 seconds, then, at that point, switch sides.

Upper Back Stretch:

Sit or stand tall with your spine straight.

Catch your hands together before you and round your upper back, coming to forward and extending your shoulder bones separated.

Hold for 15-30 seconds, feeling a stretch between your shoulder bones.

Chest Opener:

Stand tall with your feet hip-width separated.

Catch your hands behind your back and fix your arms, lifting them somewhat away from your body.

Open your chest and tenderly lift your look towards the roof.

Hold for 15-30 seconds, feeling a stretch across the front of your chest.

Forward Overlap:

Stand with your feet hip-width separated and pivot forward at your hips, bowing your knees somewhat if necessary.

Allow your chest area to hang freely towards the floor, arriving at your hands towards your feet or the ground.
Loosen up your neck and shoulders, and feel a delicate stretch along the rear of your legs and spine.
Hold for 15-30 seconds, then leisurely roll up to standing.

Situated Spinal Wind:

Sit on the floor with your legs reached out before you.
Twist your right knee and put your right foot outwardly of your left knee.
Put your left hand on your right knee and delicately bend your middle to the right, setting your right hand behind you for help.
Hold for 15-30 seconds, then, at that point, switch sides.

Kid's Posture:

Start on all fours in a tabletop position.
Sit out of sorts, arriving at your arms forward and bringing down your chest towards the floor.
Lay your temple on the ground and expand your arms out before you, feeling a delicate stretch along your back and shoulders.
Hold for 30-60 seconds, breathing profoundly into your lower back.

Conclusion:

Integrating evening extends into your everyday schedule can have significant advantages for your physical and mental prosperity. By taking a couple of seconds each night to extend and loosen up, you can deliver strain, further develop adaptability, and advance unwinding. Whether you've had a furious day or basically need to slow down before bed, these delicate activities offer a mitigating method for sustaining your body and brain. Thus, track down a peaceful space, take a couple of full breaths, and let go of the burdens of the day as you enjoy the ecstasy of night extends.

You might think that going to sleep is as easy as putting your body in bed and flipping off the lights—but just one sleepless night will probably rid you of that idea. According to the Centers for Disease Control and Prevention (CDC), one in three Americans isn't getting the sleep they need (anywhere from seven to nine hours a night). The National Sleep Foundation suggests that your body needs time to shift into sleep mode, which is why it recommends doing something relaxing before bed.

While you can certainly read, take a bath, or do something similarly relaxing, you can also do some simple stretching before bed. (Stretching isn't just for before or after a workout, after all.)

"Deep breathing and slow stretching slow the nervous system and calm the brain and body similar to meditation," says Leslie Bender, Florida-based creator of the I Am Ageless workout program and the Bender Ball, who developed the following series of six soothing stretches. Do them right before you're ready to crawl into bed to encourage sounder slumber, and pair them with lower back stretches, feet stretches, or even a morning workout to really protect and preserve your body.

1. Hip flexor opener

Stand about two to three feet from your bed, facing it. Place your right foot on the edge of the bed, bending the right knee and shifting weight forward slightly while keeping your left foot on the floor. Both feet should point forward. Reach your right arm (or both, if you want a little more challenge) toward the ceiling and hold 10 seconds, breathing deeply as you feel the muscles release. Switch sides and repeat.

2. Hamstring stretch

Stand about two to three feet from your bed, facing it. Place your right foot on bed and, keeping the leg straight, flex your right foot. With hands on hips, slowly hinge forward until you feel a stretch down the right hamstring. Without moving your body, rotate the right foot side to side eight times. Switch sides and repeat.

3. Standing spine twist

Stand about two to three feet from your bed, facing it. Reach your arms overhead so that you feel length in the front of your body. Moving from the hips, slowly lower the upper body toward the bed and place your hands on the bed. As you do this, lengthen your spine (just as you would if doing down-dog in yoga). Take your right hand off the bed and rotate the upper back to the right, reaching that arm upward while pressing into left palm. Hold for several deep breaths. Release to start and repeat other side.

4. Hip flexor stretch

Lie face-up on the bed with a rolled-up pillow under your right hip, with the leg extended on the bed. Reach your right arm overhead, thinking about lengthening through the right side of the body. Now point and flex the ankles eight times. Switch sides and repeat.

5. Spine twist

Lie face-up on the bed and bring your knees to your chest. Extend the right leg so it's resting on the bed. Place your right hand over your left hand and gently guide the left knee across your body to the right. Rotate your head left until you feel a gentle stretch in the neck. Release to start and repeat on other side.

6. Happy back

Lie face-up on the bed with a pillow under your hips. Bend your knees and them above your hips. As you bring the knees toward your chest, wrap your arms around backs of your legs. Hold at least 10 seconds, continuing to breathe deeply.

Chapter no 2
Releasing Shoulder and Neck Tension

Shoulder and neck strain are normal grumblings, particularly in the present speedy existence where a considerable lot of us go through extended periods of time sitting at work areas, slouched over PCs, or participating in dreary exercises. This strain can prompt distress, torment, and diminished versatility, influencing our general prosperity. Nonetheless, there are viable procedures and methods that can assist with easing this pressure and advance unwinding. In this complete aide, we'll investigate different strategies for delivering shoulder and neck pressure, from basic stretches to care rehearses.

Figuring out Shoulder and Neck Strain:

Prior to digging into explicit procedures, it's fundamental to comprehend the variables that add to shoulder and neck strain. Unfortunate stance, stress, muscle irregular characteristics, tedious developments, and ergonomic issues are among the essential guilty parties. Recognizing the underlying driver of your pressure can direct you in picking the most suitable procedures for help.

Extending Activities:

Extending is one of the best ways of easing shoulder and neck pressure. Here are some straightforward stretches you can integrate into your day to day daily practice:

Neck Rolls:

Sit or stand serenely with your spine erect.
Gradually lower your jawline towards your chest, feeling a stretch along the rear of your neck.
Roll your head to one side, bringing your right ear towards your right shoulder. Hold for a couple of moments.
Roll your head back to the middle and rehash on the left side.
Keep rotating sides for a few redundancies.

Shoulder Rolls:

Stand with your feet shoulder-width separated and arms hanging freely by your sides.
Gradually roll your shoulders forward in a roundabout movement, making full pivots.
Turn around the movement, moving your shoulders in reverse.
Rehash this development for a few rounds, zeroing in on relaxing any snugness in the shoulder muscles.

Upper Trapezius Stretch:

Sit or remain with your spine erect.
Arrive at your right arm over your head and put your hand on the left half of your head, delicately pulling your head towards your right shoulder.
Hold the stretch for 15-30 seconds, feeling the stretch along the left half of your neck and shoulder.
Rehash on the opposite side.

Entryway Stretch:

Stand in an entryway with your arms outstretched and hands laying on the door jamb at shoulder level.
Step forward with one foot, permitting your chest to travel through the entryway while keeping your arms fixed.
You ought to feel a delicate stretch across the front of your shoulders and chest.
Hold the stretch for 30 seconds to a moment, then discharge.

Jawline Tucks:

Sit or remain with your spine erect.
Delicately fold your jawline towards your chest, extending the rear of your neck.
Stand firm on the footing for a couple of moments, then, at that point, discharge.
Rehash for a few redundancies, zeroing in on keeping up with legitimate arrangement.

Care and Unwinding Strategies:

Notwithstanding physical stretches, care and unwinding strategies can assist with mitigating shoulder and neck strain by diminishing pressure and advancing by and large unwinding. Here are a few practices to attempt:

Profound Relaxing:

See as an agreeable situated or lying position.

Shut your eyes and take a couple of full breaths, zeroing in on filling your lungs with air.
Breathe in leisurely through your nose, permitting your mid-region to grow.
Breathe out completely through your mouth, relinquishing any pressure or stress with every breath.
Proceed with this profound breathing example for a few minutes, permitting yourself to loosen up more profoundly with each breathe out.

Moderate Muscle Unwinding (PMR):

Find a tranquil space where you can rests serenely.
Beginning with your toes, tense the muscles in each piece of your body for a couple of moments, then, at that point, discharge and unwind.
Progressively move gradually up through your legs, midsection, chest, arms, shoulders, neck, and face, straining and loosening up each muscle bunch thus.
Really focus on the muscles in your shoulders and neck, deliberately delivering any pressure you might hold.
Proceed with this interaction until you've loosened up your whole body.

Careful Reflection:

Track down an agreeable situated position and shut your eyes.
Carry your consideration regarding your breath, seeing the impression of each breathe in and breathe out.
As contemplations or interruptions emerge, basically recognize them without judgment and tenderly return your concentration to your breath.

You can likewise concentrate on the sensations in your shoulders and neck, noticing any areas of pressure with interest and empathy.
Practice careful contemplation for a few minutes to calm the psyche and advance unwinding.

Yoga:

Yoga consolidates actual stances, breathing activities, and care practices to advance unwinding and adaptability.
Numerous yoga presents explicitly focus on the shoulders and neck, assisting with delivering pressure and further develop versatility.
Consider integrating a delicate yoga practice into your daily schedule, zeroing in on stances, for example, Kid's Posture, Feline Cow, and String the Needle.

Self-Massage:

Utilizing your hands or a back rub device, tenderly ply the muscles in your shoulders and neck to deliver pressure.
Begin with light strain and progressively increment on a case by case basis, zeroing in on areas of snugness or uneasiness.
You can likewise utilize strategies, for example, pressure point massage or trigger guide treatment toward target explicit areas of strain.

Conclusion:

Shoulder and neck strain can essentially affect your personal satisfaction, however with the right methodologies and strategies, you can track down help and advance unwinding. By integrating extending works out, care practices, and unwinding strategies into your everyday daily schedule, you can ease strain, further develop portability, and develop a more prominent feeling of prosperity. Explore different avenues regarding various strategies to find what turns out best for you, and make sure to stand by listening to your body's signs as you pursue more prominent solace and simplicity in your shoulders and neck.

Tips for Relieving Shoulder and Neck Stress

When you are experiencing neck and shoulder pain and tension related to stress, managing your stress is one of the most powerful ways to decrease your symptoms. Thankfully, there are many effective ways to address stress in life. Let's look at a few.

Physical Exercise

Physical exercise of any kind is known to reduce stress. People who exercise regularly may have lower heart rates than sedentary individuals and often have more balanced, stable moods. Just 30 minutes a day of any type of movement that you enjoy can make a difference

Meditation

Practicing mindfulness and meditation can help you learn to recognize stressful thoughts so that you can let them go and not let them dominate your life. This, in turn, can reduce stress in your body, and reduce stress-related symptoms like neck and shoulder pain.

Research backs up the power of meditation on stress relief. For example, a 2021-study found that people who participated in a 6-week mindfulness program experienced decreased levels of perceived stress, as well as increased engagement at work.8

Getting Enough Sleep

You are probably aware that getting enough sleep increases your energy levels and ability to concentrate. You are also probably cognizant of the fact that increased stress levels can make it difficult to fall asleep and stay asleep. But what you may not know is that lack of sleep in and of itself can contribute to elevated levels of stress.

Therapy

Therapy can help you deal with serious mental health conditions and help you work through traumas. But it can also help you better manage the common life stresses that all of us experience.

Most of the therapy types that help you manage stress work by making you become more mindful of your thoughts and how they affect your feelings and physical reactions to stress.

Chapter no 3
Relaxing Backbends for Stress Relief

In the speedy world we live in, stress has turned into an unavoidable piece of day to day existence. It can show truly, intellectually, and inwardly, influencing our general prosperity. One viable method for combatting pressure is through the act of yoga, explicitly backbends. Backbends open the chest and heart, yet they additionally invigorate the sensory system, delivering strain and advancing unwinding. In this thorough aide, we will investigate 10 loosening up backbends that can assist with mitigating pressure and reestablish harmony to the body and brain.

Cobra Posture (Bhujangasana):

Cobra present is a delicate backbend that extends the spine, chest, and shoulders while easing strain in the lower back. To rehearse Cobra present, begin by lying on your stomach with your palms set under your shoulders. Breathe in as you press into your palms, taking your chest off the mat while keeping your pelvis grounded. Keep your elbows near your body and look forward, extending the rear of your neck. Hold the posture for 5-10 breaths, then breathe out as you discharge down to the mat.

Sphinx Posture (Salma Bhujangasana):

Sphinx present is one more delicate backbend that assists with opening the chest and extend the spine. Start by lying on your stomach with your elbows straightforwardly under your shoulders and lower arms level on the mat. Press into your lower arms as you lift your chest and look forward, keeping your shoulders loose away from your ears. Draw in your stomach muscles to help your lower back and hold the posture for 5-10 breaths, zeroing in on developing the stretch with each breathe in.

Span Posture (Setup Band asana):

Span present is a restoring backbend that eases pressure as well as fortifies the back, gluts, and legs. Lie on your back with your knees twisted and feet hip-width separated. Press into your feet as you lift your hips towards the roof, keeping your thighs lined up with one another. Entwine your fingers under you and roll your shoulders back to open the chest. Hold the posture for 5-10 breaths, breathing profoundly into the chest and midsection.

Camel Posture (Ustrasana):

Camel present is a more profound backbend that extends the whole front of the body, including the chest, midsection, and hip flexors. Stoop on the mat with your knees hip-width separated and toes tucked under. Put your hands on your lower back for help as you breathe in and lift your chest towards the roof. Delicately curve your back, arriving at your hands towards your heels while keeping your hips stacked over your knees. Hold the posture for 5-10 breaths, then leisurely returned to a bowing position.

Fish Posture (Mats asana):

Fish present is a helpful backbend that opens the chest and throat, easing pressure in the neck and shoulders. Start by lying on your back with your legs expanded and arms resting close by your body. Press into your lower arms as you lift your chest towards the roof, making a delicate curve in your upper back. Keep the load on your elbows and not your head, permitting your neck to protract. Hold the posture for 5-10 breaths, zeroing in on profound diaphragmatic relaxing.

Pup Posture (Ottawa Shishosana):

Pup present is a loosening up backbend that extends the spine, shoulders, and arms while quieting the brain. Begin your hands and knees in a tabletop position, then, at that point, walk your hands forward as you bring down your chest towards the mat, keeping your hips stacked over your knees. Lay your brow on the mat and expand your arms forward, feeling a delicate stretch in your shoulders and upper back. Hold the posture for 5-10 breaths, giving up to gravity with each breathe out.

Upheld Fish Posture:

Upheld fish present is a variety of fish represent that offers extra help and unwinding. Sit on the mat with your knees twisted and feet level on the floor, setting a reinforce or collapsed cover behind you evenly. Gradually lower your back onto the reinforce or cover, permitting your spine to curve over the help delicately. Lay your head on the mat or on a block for added level. Shut your eyes and unwind into the posture for a few minutes, relinquishing any pressure with every breath.

Upheld Extension Posture:
Upheld span present is a supportive backbend that delicately opens the chest and loosens up the sensory system. Lie on your back with your knees twisted and feet hip-width separated, setting a block or support under your sacrum. Permit your hips to be upheld by the prop as you loosen up your arms close by your body. Shut your eyes and spotlight on your breath, giving up to the help of the prop and feeling the arrival of strain in your body.

Helpful Sphinx Posture:

Helpful Sphinx present is a profoundly loosening up backbend that advances pressure alleviation and close to home equilibrium. Start by lying on your stomach with your elbows bowed and lower arms laying on the mat, framing a delicate curve in your upper back. Place a reinforce or collapsed cover under your chest for help, permitting your heart to dissolve towards the earth. Shut your eyes and inhale profoundly into the posture, giving up to the impression of opening and extension with every breath.

Leaning back Bound Point Posture (Sputa Buddha Kona Sana):

Leaning back bound point present is a supportive backbend that opens the chest and hips while quieting the psyche. Lie on your back with your knees bowed and feet together, permitting your knees to drop out to the sides in a butterfly shape. Place a reinforce or collapsed cover under your spine in an upward direction for help, permitting your chest to open tenderly. Rest your arms close by your body with palms looking up, shutting your eyes and giving up to the posture for a few minutes.

Conclusion:

Integrating these 10 loosening up backbends into your yoga practice can be a successful method for decreasing pressure and advance unwinding. Whether you're searching for a delicate stretch or a more profound delivery, these postures offer different choices to suit your requirements. Make sure to pay attention to your body and practice with mindfulness, permitting yourself to relinquish strain and discover a sense of reconciliation inside. By making backbends a customary piece of your daily practice, you can develop a feeling of quiet and equilibrium that reaches out a long ways past the yoga mat.

Camel Pose

Camel pose may be tricky, but it's worth a try for the way it relieves stress. "As a backbend, it helps to open up your chest and encourages the release of pent-up emotions, energy, or stress," Passalacqua explains. "It can also help stretch your chest and back if you hunch your posture while stressed."

- Kneel on your yoga mat.

- Keep your knees hip-width apart and the rest of your body upright.

- As you inhale, raise your chest and arch your back while keeping your thighs straight up.

- Keep leaning back until you can place the palms of your hands on your heels, if possible.

- Allow your head to tilt back until you're facing the ceiling.

- Hold for 30 to 60 seconds.

Seated Forward Fold

When you're stressed, tension starts to build up in your shoulders, back, hips, and hamstrings. By purposefully releasing these areas with a seated forward fold, Passalacqua says it can promote feelings of comfort and mindfulness.

- Sit on your yoga mat.

- Extend your legs straight out in front of you.

- Lift your arms and point them toward the ceiling.

- Fold from your hips, bringing your torso over your legs.

- Stretch through the length of your back rather than hunching to reach your toes.

- Hold your legs or grab your feet with your hands, depending on how far you can reach.

- Hold for one to two minutes as you breathe.

Chapter no 4
Hip Openers for Releasing Emotions

In the excursion of comprehensive prosperity, the association between the body and psyche is unquestionable. Our actual stance, developments, and even pressures held inside our muscles frequently mirror our profound state. Among the different locales of the body where feelings can become held up, the hips stand apart as an especially huge area of capacity. Whether it's because of delayed sitting, stress, or unsettled feelings, pressure in the hips can limit our development and repress profound delivery. In any case, through the act of hip-opening activities, we can disentangle these bunches, free caught feelings, and encourage a more profound feeling of physical and close to home opportunity. In this far reaching guide, we'll investigate the connection between the hips and feelings and dig into different hip-opening activities pointed toward working with profound delivery.

Figuring out the Hips-Feelings Association:

The hips are frequently alluded to as the body's "garbage cabinet" for feelings. This is on the grounds that the hips will more often than not collect pressure and snugness, going about as a stockpiling unit for unsettled sentiments and stress. Different elements add to this peculiarity:

Stationary Way of life:

In the present stationary society, a considerable lot of us spend delayed periods sitting, whether at work areas, in vehicles, or on lounge chairs. This consistent sitting abbreviates the hip flexors and makes strain in the encompassing muscles, prompting solidness and profound stagnation.

Stress and Injury:

Feelings like apprehension, nervousness, and bitterness can appear as actual pressure in the hips. Moreover, horrendous encounters might make people subliminally contract their hip muscles as a type of security, prompting constant snugness.

Fiery Blockages:

As indicated by different comprehensive practices, for example, yoga and Customary Chinese Medication, the hips are related with the Sad his Thana (sacral) chakra, which oversees feelings, innovativeness, and arousing quality. Fiery blockages in this space can upset the progression of feelings and frustrate self-articulation.

By tending to these elements through designated hip opening activities, we can start to deliver repressed feelings and reestablish harmony to both body and brain.

Hip-Opening Activities for Close to home Delivery:

Pigeon Posture (Eke Padas Raja kapotasana):

This yoga present focuses on the hip flexors, gluts, and performs, delivering well established pressure in the hips. As you sink into the posture, center around profound, diaphragmatic breathing to work with the arrival of feelings put away in the pelvis.

Butterfly Posture (Buddha Kona Sana):

Sitting on the floor, bring the bottoms of your feet together and let your knees fall open to the sides. Tenderly press your knees toward the ground while keeping your spine long. This posture extends the inward thighs and crotch, advancing profound delivery and give up.

Low Lurch (Anjaneyasana):

Stage one foot forward into a jump position, keeping the back knee on the ground. Sink your hips down and forward, feeling a stretch in the hip flexors of the back leg. Permit any feelings that emerge to be recognized without judgment as you hold the posture.

Frog Posture:

From a tabletop position, spread your knees wide while keeping your lower legs in accordance with your knees. Gradually lower your hips toward the ground, feeling a profound stretch in the internal thighs and crotch. This posture can be serious, so pay attention to your body and inhale profoundly through any distress.

Hip Circles:

Stand with your feet hip-width separated and hands on your hips. Start to make slow circles with your hips, zeroing in on smooth, smooth motions. As you circle your hips, envision working up and delivering stale feelings put away in the pelvis.

Upheld Extension Posture:

Lie on your back with your knees twisted and feet hip-width separated. Place a block or reinforce under your sacrum and permit your hips to unwind onto the help. Shut your eyes and inhale profoundly, imagining strain liquefying away from your hips and pelvis.

Conclusion:

Feelings are not simply bound to the domain of the brain; they are profoundly interwoven with our actual bodies. By integrating hip-opening activities into our health schedules, we can take advantage of the body's insight and delivery put away feelings. Whether through yoga, extending, or careful development, the freedom of our hips can prompt more prominent profound opportunity and by and large prosperity. Make sure to move toward these activities with persistence, empathy, and a readiness to embrace anything that feelings might emerge en route. As you open your hips, you open yourself to a more profound comprehension and acknowledgment of your internal world.

Four exercises to open the hips and lengthen your muscles:
1. Pigeon pose

A popular yoga pose offering a deep stretch across the thighs, back, groin, performs, and psoas. The easiest way to get into the Pigeon Pose is by starting in a Downward Dog position or on your hands and knees.

You may place padding or a folded blanket under your hip to make this pose more comfortable. You can slowly enter a forward bend when you get into the pose. Focus on your breathing and the different sensations that arise emotional, mental, or physical.
 even this unplanned activity and accomplishments took us closer to our purpose.

There are often clues to learning in the small moments when we do unexpected things steering us down uncertain roads. And finding these are like finding gold which teaches us about embracing and avoiding certain activities and decisions in the future.

Other questions:

The questions above a are a minimal set to consider in a reflection practice. As you discover more about your purpose you may change, or add questions to your own practice.

Other questions I sometimes add are:

Was I the role model for others that I want to be?

This question is a beautiful one to consider if we are in roles of leadership or influence. It inquires about how we show up to those who look up to us and pattern their behavior.

A great leader serves through leading by example.

So what is the role model you want to be?

And how will you show up for those who look up to you?

What three things am I grateful for on this day?

As humans, we are not very good at being grateful. Sometimes the big moments connect us to gratitude, but we often miss the small moments.

Consciously creating a moment in our reflection to focus on appreciation connects us daily with what we are grateful for, whether those things or people have large or small impacts in our lives.

In addition, there is scientific evidence that gratitude has benefits for our health and wellbeing.

If I could have today over again, what three things could I do to make it even better?

This question is one of my favorite ones to reflect on. Of course, it carries within it the presupposition that I have had a great day, but it also opens up the possibility that, had I done something else, something more, it could be even better.

This question leads us down the path of innovation, the way of looking for something new, novel and different. And it suggests options which can make any future day better.

Optional Step Five: Journal about your practice

Journaling is not compulsory, but it serves to preserve a record of reflective thinking. Over time it shows the paths you took on your journey to purpose, and it highlights the opportunities and ideas that come from deep thought.

On many occasions, when I face a mountain that seems too steep to climb, I find solace, courage, and motivation in my journals, whether it be missteps, bumbling approaches or incredible insights.

A carefully kept journal is a measure of personal growth and a foundation for achievement.
 The journey to living your purpose is on a road that leads inwards. Reflection comes from roots of curiosity and fascination with what is possible for you and shines a mirror on the wisdom of the best version you want to

be. A daily reflection practice will chart a path to the future and, like the captain of a ship, correct the course to end up where you want to be.

Give yourself the gift of reflection and embrace a journey that leads to fulfillment, joy and happiness!

2. Lizard Pose

The lizard pose, also known as the gecko pose, focuses on the hips, groin, and inner hamstrings. This pose provides an intense stretch, but we recommend trying a variation if you're still building up your flexibility. If you enjoyed the lizard pose, a similar hip-opening pose to try is a low lunge. Once again, Downward-Facing Dog provides a suitable place to start. When you're ready, step one foot up to the outside of your hand. Ensure your knee is at a 90-degree angle and positioned above the ankle. Hold this pose for a few slow deep breaths before repeating it on the other side.

. Reclining twist

This next pose (also referred to as the Supine Spinal Twist) is ideal for releasing stress as it targets the gluts, chest, and oblique. This pose doesn't focus on the hips as much as the others but provides a 'heart opening' position.

rinse the body

Many use this pose alongside hip openers to "rinse" the body and allow emotions to flow. To deepen this stretch and make it work for you, ensure you're not holding your breath. Instead, breathe deeply and accept where your body is in this position, whether your knee makes it to the floor or not.

4. Seated butterfly

This last stretch offers a final cleansing movement for your hips. Start in a seat with your spine straight and your shoulders relaxed. By bringing the soles of the feet together, opening up your legs, and letting gravity pull your knees down, your hips receive a deep, slow stretch. The Butterfly Stretch will target the inner thighs, hips, lower back, and groin. Do not force your legs down; instead, let them open gently as you focus on deep breathing.

Closing thoughts

Hip-opening stretches provide a deeply nurturing way to care for the body, improve mobility, and boost energy. Hip openers may also release suppressed emotion and clear energy blocks.

Chapter no 5
Calming Twist to Aid Digestion

In the buzzing about of present day life, our stomach related framework frequently endures the worst part of pressure, sporadic dietary patterns, and unfortunate food decisions. Integrating quieting turns into your routine can give alleviation not exclusively to your body yet additionally for your brain. These delicate yoga presents help in processing as well as advance unwinding, assisting you with tracking down balance in the midst of the mayhem of regular day to day existence. In this complete aide, we will investigate 20 quieting turns that can uphold your stomach related wellbeing and upgrade your general prosperity.

Situated Spinal Turn (Arch Matsyendrasana):

Begin in a situated situation with your legs expanded.
Twist your right knee and put your right foot outwardly of your left knee.
Put your left elbow outwardly of your right knee and tenderly wind your middle to the right.
Hold the posture for a few breaths, then, at that point, rehash on the opposite side.

Recumbent Spinal Turn (Sputa Matsyendrasana):

Lie on your back with your arms reached out to the sides.
Twist your knees and bring them towards your chest.

Drop your knees to the right side while keeping your shoulders grounded.
Hold the posture for a couple of breaths, then, at that point, switch sides.

String the Needle Posture (Persia Balsams):

Start on all fours in a tabletop position.
Slide your right arm under your left arm, bringing down your right shoulder and ear to the mat.
Press into your passed close by to extend the contort.
Hold for a few breaths, then, at that point, switch sides.

Spun Triangle Posture (Parivrtta Trikonasana):

Begin in a standing situation with your feet about hip-width separated.
Step your left foot back and turn it out at a 45-degree point.
Stretch out your arms out to the sides and reach forward with your right hand.
Bring down your right hand to the beyond your left foot or a block, and wind your middle to the left.
Hold the posture for a couple of breaths, then, at that point, rehash on the opposite side.

Rotated Seat Posture (Parivrtta Utkatasana):

Start in a standing situation with your feet together.

Twist your knees and lower your hips into a squat position, as though you were sitting in a nonexistent seat.
Unite your hands at your heart place.
Bend your middle to the right, snaring your left elbow outwardly of your right thigh.
Hold for a few breaths, then, at that point, switch sides.

Rotated Side Point Posture (Parivrtta Parsvakonasana):

Begin in a thrust position with your right foot forward and your left foot back.
Twist your right knee and lower into a lurch, keeping your left leg straight and solid.
Put your left hand on the mat or a block within your right foot.
Broaden your right arm up towards the roof and afterward bend your middle to one side, arriving at your right arm over your head.
Hold for a couple of breaths, then, at that point, switch sides.

Wound Reptile Posture (Parivrtta Utahan Pristhasana):

Start in a low lurch position with your right foot forward and your left knee on the mat.
Put your hands within your right foot.
Bring down your passed on lower arm to the mat and turn your middle to one side, arriving at your right arm up towards the roof.
Hold for a few breaths, then switch sides.

Situated Ahead Curve Contort (Paschimottanasana Turn):

Sit on the floor with your legs stretched out before you.
Twist your right knee and put your right foot outwardly of your left thigh.
Arrive at your left arm up towards the roof and afterward turn your middle to the right, carrying your passed on elbow to the beyond your right knee.
Hold for a couple of breaths, then switch sides.

Bent Seat Posture (Parivrtta Utkatasana):

Start in a standing situation with your feet together.
Twist your knees and lower your hips into a squat position, as though you were sitting in a nonexistent seat.
Unite your hands at your heart place.
Turn your middle to the right, snaring your left elbow outwardly of your right thigh.
Hold for a few breaths, then, at that point, switch sides.

Rotated Half Moon Posture (Parivrtta Arch Chandra Sana):

Begin in a standing situation with your feet together.
Twist forward and put your right hand on the mat or a block.
Lift your left advantage towards the roof, coming into a half moon present.
Broaden your left arm up towards the roof and afterward curve your middle to one side, arriving at your left arm over your head.

Hold for a couple of breaths, then, at that point, switch sides.

Spun Head-to-Knee Posture (Parivrtta Jana Sirs asana):

Sit on the floor with your legs stretched out before you.
Twist your right knee and spot the underside of your right foot against your left internal thigh.
Arrive at your right arm behind you and put your right hand on the mat.
Breathe in to protract your spine, then breathe out and curve your middle to one side, arriving at your left arm up towards the roof.
Hold for a few breaths, then switch sides.

Bent Expanded Side Point Posture (Parivrtta Outhit Parsvakonasana):

Begin in a lurch position with your right foot forward and your left foot back.
Broaden your right leg and lower your right hand to the mat or a block outwardly of your right foot.
Arrive at your left arm up towards the roof and afterward curve your middle to the right, arriving at your left arm over your head.
Hold for a couple of breaths, then, at that point, switch sides.

Bent High Rush (Parivrtta Arch Uttanasana):

Start in a high thrust position with your right foot forward and your left foot back.

Put your hands on your hips and square your hips to the front of the mat.

Breathe in to extend your spine, then breathe out and wind your middle to the right, carrying your passed on elbow to the beyond your right knee.

Hold for a few breaths, then switch sides.

Situated Bend (Marichyasana):

Sit on the floor with your legs reached out before you.

Twist your right knee and put your right foot outwardly of your left thigh.

Breathe in to extend your spine, then, at that point, breathe out and curve your middle to the right, carrying your passed available to the beyond your right knee and your right hand behind you.

Hold for a couple of breaths, then, at that point, switch sides.

Rotated Sickle Rush (Parivrtta Anjaneyasana):

Start in a low lurch position with your right foot forward and your left knee on the mat.

Breathe in to lift your middle upstanding, then breathe out and bend your middle to the right, arriving at your left arm forward and your right arm back.

Hold for a few breaths, then switch sides.

Rotated Side Board Posture (Parivrtta Vasisthasana):

Begin in a side board position with your right hand on the mat and your feet stacked.

Breathe in to lift your left arm up towards the roof, then breathe out and wind your middle to the right, arriving at your left arm under your body.

Hold for a couple of breaths, then, at that point, switch sides.

Rotated Wide-Legged Forward Curve (Parivrtta Parasite Padottanasana):

Stand with your feet wide separated and lined up with one another.

Breathe in to extend your spine, then, at that point, breathe out and crease forward from your hips, carrying your hands to the mat or a block.

Breathe in to lift your middle mostly, then, at that point, breathe out and bend your middle to the right, arriving at your left arm up towards the roof.

Hold for a few breaths, then, at that point, switch sides.

Spun Half Ruler of the Fishes Posture (Parivrtta Arch Matsyendrasana):

Sit on the floor with your legs reached out before you.

Twist your right knee and put your right foot outwardly of your left thigh.

Breathe in to protract your spine, then, at that point, breathe out and turn your middle to the right, carrying your passed on elbow to the beyond your right knee.

Hold for a couple of breaths, then switch sides.

Rotated Camel Posture (Parivrtta Ustrasana):

Stoop on the mat with your knees hip-width separated and your thighs opposite to the floor.

Put your hands on your lower back with your fingers pointing down.
Breathe in to lift your chest and curve your back, then, at that point, breathe out and turn your middle to the right, arriving at your left hand towards your right heel.
Hold for a few breaths, then switch sides.

Situated Half Spinal Wind (Arch Matsyendrasana):

Sit on the floor with your legs reached out before you.
Twist your right knee and put your right foot outwardly of your left thigh.
Breathe in to protract your spine, then breathe out and curve your middle to the right, carrying your passed on elbow to the beyond your right knee.
Hold for a couple of breaths, then, at that point, switch sides.

Conclusion:

These quieting turns offer actual advantages for absorption as well as mental unwinding, assisting with calming the anxieties of day to day existence. Integrate these postures into your yoga practice routinely to help your stomach related wellbeing and advance generally speaking prosperity. Make sure to pay attention to your body and inhale profoundly as you travel through each posture, permitting yourself to discover a sense of harmony and tranquility in both body and brain.

1. Seated Twist (Arch Matsyendrasana)

This gentle twisting posture helps stimulate digestion and alleviate symptoms associated with IBS. Twisting the abdominal region provides a gentle massage to the internal organs, including the intestines, which can help regulate bowel movements and relieve constipation or bloating.

Start by sitting on the floor with your legs extended. Cross your right leg over your left and place your left hand behind you for support. Twist your torso to the left, placing your right hand on your left knee. Hold the pose for 30 seconds to 1 minute, breathing deeply. Repeat on the other side by crossing your left leg over your right knee and twisting to the right.

2. Cat-Cow pose (Marjaryasana-Bitilasana)

This pose involves gentle and rhythmic spine movements, which help stimulate digestion and can alleviate symptoms of IBS. The Cat-Cow pose alternates between arching the back upward (Cow pose) and rounding the back downward (Cat pose), effectively massaging the abdominal region and encouraging healthy bowel motility.

Start on your hands and knees with your hands placed under your shoulders and your knees under your hips. Inhale and gently drop your belly towards the floor, arching your back and lifting your head, creating a gentle backbend. Exhale and round your spine upward, tucking your chin towards your chest and engaging your abdominal muscles. Flow between these two positions, repeating the movements for several breaths.

3. Child's Pose (Balsams)

This gentle posture helps to calm the mind and relax the body. The Child's Pose provides gentle compression to the abdominal region, promoting relaxation and relieving tension in the gut.

Start by kneeling on the floor with your knees hip-width apart. Sit back on your heels and slowly lower your torso, bending forward from the hips. Extend your arms forward, allowing them to rest on the floor before you with your palms facing down. As you fold forward, gently rest your forehead on the mat or turn your head to one side, whichever is more comfortable. Relax your shoulders, release tension, and let your body sink into the pose. Breathe deeply, focusing on the expansion of your back and the relaxation of your entire body. Stay in this position for as long as it feels comfortable.

4. Bridge pose (Setup Band asana)

This backbend posture helps stimulate the digestive system and alleviate symptoms of IBS. By lifting the pelvis and arching the spine, the Bridge pose gently massages the abdominal organs, improving digestion and promoting bowel regularity. The bridge pose opens up the chest, increasing lung capacity and encouraging deep breathing, activating the parasympathetic nervous system and calming the digestive system.

Lie flat on your back with your knees bent and feet flat on the floor, hip-width apart. Place your arms alongside your body, palms facing down. Inhale deeply, and as you exhale slowly, press your feet into the ground, engaging your gluts and lifting your hips off the floor. Keep your thighs and feet parallel to each other. Interlace your fingers beneath your body and roll your shoulders to open your chest. If it's more comfortable, you can keep your hands flat on the mat instead. Hold the pose for a few deep breaths, maintaining a steady rhythm.

5. Corpse pose (Svanasana)

This pose completely relaxes the body and mind, encouraging deep rest and rejuvenation. Stress and anxiety often exacerbate IBS symptoms, and Svanasana helps reduce these factors. Lying down on your back with arms and legs extended allows the body to fully relax and release tension. This pose promotes a state of calm and relaxation, reducing stress levels and promoting better digestion.

Chapter no 6
Soothing Forward Folds for Relaxation

In the hustle and bustle of modern life, finding moments of tranquility is essential for our mental and physical well-being. Yoga, an ancient practice originating in India, offers a pathway to relaxation and inner peace. Among the many yoga poses, forward folds stand out as particularly effective for calming the mind, releasing tension, and promoting relaxation. In this comprehensive guide, we will explore various soothing forward folds, their benefits, and techniques to enhance your practice. Whether you're a seasoned yogi or a beginner, these poses can help you unwind and rejuvenate.

Understanding Forward Folds:

Forward folds, also known as Uttanasana in Sanskrit, involve bending forward from the hips, lengthening the spine, and bringing the torso closer to the legs. This action stretches the entire back body, including the spine, hamstrings, and calves. Forward folds also calm the nervous system, relieve stress, and encourage introspection.

Benefits of Forward Folds:

Stress Relief:

 Forward folds stimulate the parasympathetic nervous system, which promotes relaxation and reduces stress levels.

Improved Posture: Regular practice of forward folds helps lengthen the spine and release tension in the back, leading to improved posture.

Enhanced Flexibility: Consistent practice of forward folds gradually increases flexibility in the hamstrings, hips, and lower back.

Digestive Health: The gentle compression of the abdomen in forward folds stimulates digestion and can alleviate symptoms of bloating and constipation.

Emotional Release: Forward folds create space in the body, allowing for the release of stored emotions and mental tension.

Preparing for Forward Folds:

Warm-Up: It's essential to prepare the body before diving into deep forward folds. Start with gentle warm-up poses like Cat-Cow, Downward-Facing Dog, and Sun Salutations to awaken the muscles and loosen the joints.

Breath Awareness: Pay attention to your breath throughout the practice. Deep, steady breathing helps relax the body and quiet the mind, making the forward fold experience more soothing.

Props: Props such as blocks, straps, and bolsters can support your forward fold practice, especially if you're working on flexibility or have any physical limitations.

Soothing Forward Fold Sequences:

Standing Forward Fold (Uttanasana): This foundational pose can be practiced with feet hip-width apart or together. Allow the upper body to relax completely over the legs, releasing tension in the spine and hamstrings.

Seated Forward Fold (Paschimottanasana):
Sitting on the floor, extend the legs forward and fold forward from the hips. Keep the spine long and avoid

rounding the back excessively. Use props like a strap to reach the feet if necessary.

Wide-Legged Forward Fold (Parasite Padottanasana):

Stand with legs wide apart and fold forward, keeping the spine extended. This pose offers a deep stretch to the hamstrings and inner thighs.

Supported Forward Fold:

Place a bolster or folded blanket on the floor and lie down with the torso supported. Relax completely into the prop, allowing gravity to deepen the stretch without strain.

Supine Forward Fold (Sputa Padangusthasana):

Lie on your back and draw one knee towards the chest, holding onto the big toe with a strap. Extend the leg upward, keeping the other leg grounded. This pose stretches the hamstrings and relaxes the lower back.

Seated Forward Fold with Twist:

From a seated position, fold forward and then add a gentle twist to one side, placing the opposite hand on the outer edge of the foot or on the floor. Twisting enhances the spinal rotation and releases tension in the back.

Tips for Deepening Your Forward Fold Practice:

Patience and Persistence: Flexibility takes time to develop, so be patient with yourself and practice consistently.

Listen to Your Body: Honor your body's limitations and avoid pushing into pain or discomfort. Respect your edge and breathe into the stretch gradually.

Incorporate Props: Experiment with different props to find what supports your body best in forward folds. Props can make the poses more accessible and enjoyable.

Relaxation Techniques:

 Incorporate relaxation techniques such as visualization, mindfulness, or gentle music to enhance the soothing effects of forward folds.

Modify as Needed:

 Modify the poses as needed to accommodate any injuries or physical limitations. Remember that yoga is about finding balance and harmony in your body, mind, and spirit.

Conclusion:

Soothing forward folds offer a sanctuary of calm in the midst of life's demands. By integrating these poses into your yoga practice, you can cultivate relaxation, release tension, and nourish your overall well-being. Whether you practice for a few minutes each day or dedicate longer sessions to your forward fold practice, may you find solace and serenity in each gentle bend forward. As you journey deeper into the practice of yoga, may you discover the profound peace that resides within.

By embracing the transformative power of forward folds, you embark on a journey of self-discovery and inner peace. Let each fold forward be an invitation to surrender, to let go, and to connect with the essence of your being. In the stillness of the pose, may you find the whispers of your soul and the wisdom of your heart.

Sit on the floor with your legs extended in front of you.

Press down through the backs of the thighs and extend through your heels, flexing the toes.

Press your palms or fingertips into the floor beside your hips to lengthen the spine.

Draw the navel up and in and lift the bottom ribs away from the hips.

Lean forward from the hip joints, not the waist.

Keep the spine long as the torso bows forward over the legs.

Place hands on shins, ankles, outside of the feet or on the floor alongside the legs.

With each inhale, lift and lengthen the spine, drawing the chest forward.

With each exhale release a little more fully into the forward bend.

Allow the lower belly, ribs and then chest to rest on the tops of the thighs.

Stay in this pose for 5-10 breaths.

To exit, extend the chest forward and inhale as you come up with a long spine.

Tips for Mastering Seated Forward Fold Pose
If you are new to seated forward fold, take it slow. Most of us have tight hips and hamstrings and it might be challenging enough just to sit up straight with legs extended.

Use props or modify as needed…sit on a yoga blanket to create more space at the hips or bend the knees to relieve any hamstring strain. Use a yoga strap around the feet rather than hands.

Do not pull or force your way into a deeper bend but think about lengthening and releasing to deepen the pose.

Avoid locking the knees by engaging the quadriceps. If you tend to hyper-extend at the knee joints, micro-bend the knees in the pose.

Release shoulders away from the ears and soften the shoulder blades down the back.

Relax your jaw, face, and neck as you fold forward. Flutter the lips or sigh to release tension in the jaw, neck and shoulders.

Chapter no 7
Grounding Meditation for inner peace

In the hurrying around of present day life, discovering a true sense of reconciliation can some of the time feel like a far off dream. In the midst of the disorder of everyday obligations and outer stressors, fundamental to develop rehearses help us reconnect with ourselves and track down peacefulness inside. One strong method for accomplishing internal harmony is through establishing reflection. Establishing contemplation includes fixating your mindfulness on the current second, interfacing with the earth, and quieting the psyche. In this aide, we'll investigate a far reaching establishing contemplation practice intended to bring you profound unwinding and internal serenity.

Grasping Establishing:

Establishing Characterized: What's the significance here to be grounded? Investigating the idea of establishing and its importance for mental, profound, and otherworldly prosperity.

The Significance of Establishing:

Examining the advantages of establishing, including pressure decrease, expanded mindfulness, close to home soundness, and improved lucidity of brain.

How Establishing Functions:

Making sense of the standards behind establishing reflection, for example, mooring to the current second, associating with nature, and adjusting energy.

Planning for Establishing Contemplation:

Making a Holy Space:

Ways to set up a peaceful climate helpful for contemplation, including choosing a calm area, designing with normal components, and utilizing fragrance based treatment.

Open to Seating:

Picking an open to guest plan to help your reflection practice, whether it's sitting leg over leg on a pad, utilizing a contemplation seat, or sitting in a seat with appropriate stance.

Setting Goals:

Explaining your goals for the reflection meeting, like looking for internal harmony, delivering pressure, or developing care.

Establishing Strategies:

Careful Relaxing: Directed practice on careful breathing to moor your mindfulness right now and quiet the psyche.

Body Sweep:

Bit by bit directions for a body examine contemplation, zeroing in on each piece of the body to deliver strain and advance unwinding.

Visualization:

Utilizing representation methods to envision roots reaching out from your body into the earth, establishing you to the world's energy and strength.

Nature Association:

Investigating strategies for interfacing with nature during contemplation, for example, imagining normal scenes, paying attention to nature sounds, or rehearsing open air reflection.

Developing Your Training:

Integrating Certifications:

Coordinating good confirmations into your establishing reflection to build up sensations of internal harmony, strength, and flexibility.

Appreciation Practice:

Developing appreciation during contemplation by pondering things you're thankful for in your life, encouraging a feeling of satisfaction and overflow.

Journaling: Journaling prompts to think about your establishing contemplation experience, including bits of knowledge acquired, feelings felt, and regions for development.

Moderate Unwinding:

High level strategy for moderate muscle unwinding to extend unwinding and discharge further layers of strain from the body.

Coordinating Establishing into Day to day existence:

Careful Development: Investigating careful development practices like yoga, Jujitsu, or strolling reflection as ways of remaining grounded over the course of the day.

Establishing Ceremonies:

Making every day establishing customs to moor yourself right now and keep a feeling of inward harmony in the midst of day to day exercises.

Self-Compassion: Rehearsing self-empathy and taking care of oneself as fundamental parts of establishing, supporting yourself with generosity and understanding.

Keeping up with Consistency: Methods for integrating establishing contemplation into your everyday daily schedule and conquering normal deterrents to consistency.

Conclusion:

Establishing reflection offers a pathway to inward harmony and close to home versatility in an undeniably tumultuous world. By developing a customary establishing practice, you can reconnect with your actual pith, track down comfort in the midst of life's difficulties, and experience a significant feeling of peacefulness. Keep in mind, the excursion to internal harmony is progressing, however with commitment and practice, you can secure yourself right now and explore existence with beauty and poise.

Inner Peace Fellowship Meditation (IPF Meditation) comes from the Vedic tradition of India, which is over 3,000 years old. IPF Meditation uses the same Sanskrit mantras that yogis in India have been using and refining for thousands of years. IPF Meditation is very easy to learn, and you can get many valuable benefits from practicing it. Millions of people in 235 countries and jurisdictions have used these meditation instructions.

You learn to meditate by meditating. The silence and stillness you experience in meditation and the increased happiness and diminished stress you experience outside meditation are so attractive and welcomed that you naturally teach yourself how to go deeper into that silence and stillness each time you meditate.

Daily Practice of Meditation

Meditate every morning and every evening for 15-30 minutes. Use your mantra in Your First Meditation above. It is best to meditate before you eat. Try to meditate in a quiet place but if you do not have a quiet place to meditate that is okay. Noise is not a barrier to meditating.

Sit quietly, close your eyes, and do nothing for a minute or so. Thoughts will come and that is okay. It is natural to have thoughts during meditation. After a minute or so, in the same natural way that thoughts come, and without moving your tongue or lips, quietly inside start saying your mantra. Slowly repeat your mantra until you are done meditating. When thoughts come, gently return to saying your mantra. When you finish meditating, lay down and rest for 4-5 minutes.

At times you may be saying your mantra unclearly, and that is okay. At times you may not be saying your mantra at all, and instead your mantra may be a sense or a feeling of your mantra, and that is okay. At times all thoughts and your mantra may disappear and you may simply be aware, and that is okay.

You may go to sleep during meditation, and that is okay. When you wake up after being asleep, meditate for a few more minutes and then lay down and rest for 4-5 minutes.

1. Enjoy a natural high as the release of endorphins associated with meditation allows you to relax and de-stress from daily challenges.

2. Enjoy the elevated well-being associated with whole-brain functioning like improved decision making and enhanced ability to concentrate.

3. Build a bridge between the logical, analytical capabilities of your brain's left hemisphere and the imaginative, intuitive ones of the right, expanding creativity, flow and productivity.

4. Achieve greater objectivity and perspective that can help you maintain calm in all situations.

5. Tap into deeper states of consciousness where you will enjoy inner stillness, harmony and balance in your physical, emotional and mental dimensions.

7. Reduce your unconscious reactions to people and events that trigger an emotional response; reactions that trap you in past anger or future anxiety and keep you from enjoying the present moment.

8. Expand your emotional clearing process and release energy for more enjoyable pursuits.

9. Enjoy higher levels of wellness as reduced stress levels promote healthier bodies, emotions and minds.

10. Increase self-love, acceptance, and happiness.

Chapter no 8
Restorative yoga for Deep Relaxation

In the hurrying around of present day life, finding snapshots of profound unwinding can feel like an extravagance. Be that as it may, focusing on unwinding is fundamental for keeping up with physical, mental, and profound prosperity. Helpful yoga offers a pathway to this unwinding by using delicate postures, steady props, and cognizant breathing strategies to initiate a condition of profound smoothness and reclamation. In this aide, we will investigate the standards and practices of helpful yoga, its advantages, key postures, and ways to integrate it into your daily schedule for profound unwinding.

Grasping Helpful Yoga:

Helpful yoga is a delicate and remedial type of yoga that spotlights on unwinding and restoration. In contrast to additional dynamic styles of yoga, for example, Vinyasa or Astana, which underline development and strength building, helpful yoga urges professionals to unwind profoundly into upheld models for broadened periods. The essential objective is to initiate the parasympathetic sensory system, otherwise called the "rest and condensation" reaction, which checks the pressure reaction of the thoughtful sensory system.

Advantages of Helpful Yoga:

The advantages of helpful yoga stretch out past actual unwinding to envelop mental and close to home prosperity. A portion of the key advantages include:

Stress Decrease:

Supportive yoga sets off the unwinding reaction, assisting with decreasing pressure chemicals like cortisol and advance a feeling of serenity and peacefulness.

Further developed Rest Quality:

Normal act of supportive yoga can assist with further developing rest quality by loosening up the body and quieting the brain, making it simpler to nod off and stay unconscious over the course of the evening.

Improved Adaptability:

While helpful yoga may not include extraordinary extending like different types of yoga, holding delicate postures with the backing of props can steadily further develop adaptability and scope of movement after some time.

Close to home Recuperating:

The reflective part of supportive yoga permits specialists to develop care and mindfulness, which can work with profound mending and strength.

Key Standards of Supportive Yoga:

Support: The utilization of props like supports, covers, blocks, and lashes is fundamental to helpful yoga. Props offer help and solace, permitting the body to unwind profoundly into each posture without strain or exertion.

Comfort: In supportive yoga, solace is focused on over exertion. Postures ought to be changed depending on the situation to guarantee that the body feels upheld and loose.

Mindfulness:

Rehearsing care is fundamental in supportive yoga. By carrying attention to the breath, sensations in the body, and contemplations in the psyche, specialists can extend their unwinding experience.

Duration:

Helpful yoga presents are commonly held for longer lengths, going from 5 to 20 minutes or more. This lengthy hold permits the body and brain to settle profoundly into unwinding.

Key Postures in Supportive Yoga:

Upheld Youngster's Posture (Balsams):

This delicate forward twist extends the hips, thighs, and lower back while advancing a feeling of give up and deliver. Backing can be furnished with a support or stacked covers put under the middle.

Upheld Leaning back Bound Point Posture (Sputa Buddha Kona Sana):

This helpful posture opens the hips and chest while advancing unwinding and internal quiet. Props, for example, reinforces or collapsed covers can be put under the knees and middle for help.

Advantages the-Wall Posture (Vicariate Karana):

This reversal present advances flow, eases expanding in the legs, and prompts a feeling of unwinding. A reinforce or collapsed cover can be put under the hips for added help.

Upheld Carcass Posture (Svanasana):

The last unwinding present in any yoga practice, Svanasana is particularly helpful when upheld with props like reinforces under the knees and a sweeping under the head.

Integrating Helpful Yoga into Your Daily schedule:

To encounter the advantages of supportive yoga, consider integrating it into your every day or week after week schedule. Here are a few ways to get everything rolling:

Establish a Loosening up Climate:

Find a peaceful, agreeable space liberated from interruptions where you can rehearse helpful yoga without interference.

Accumulate Props:

Put resources into a couple of yoga props like reinforces, covers, blocks, and lashes to help your supportive practice.

Put away Opportunity:

Plan committed time for supportive yoga practice, regardless of whether it's only a couple of moments every day. Consistency is vital to encountering the full advantages.

Pay attention to Your Body:

Focus on how your body feels in each posture and change on a case by case basis to guarantee solace and unwinding.

Conclusion:

Supportive yoga offers a strong remedy to the burdens of current life, giving a safe-haven to profound unwinding and revival. By embracing the standards of help, solace, care, and term, you can open the groundbreaking capability of this delicate yet significant practice. Whether you're looking for help from pressure, better rest, expanded adaptability, or close to home recuperating, supportive yoga offers a pathway to all encompassing prosperity. Begin your excursion towards profound unwinding today, and find the harmony that dwells inside.

Deeply relax with as your body is completely supported in longer held yoga poses

Restorative yoga enables deep relaxation as you holding poses for longer periods of time with the help of props to completely support you.

The main focus of Restorative Yoga is that by relaxing in poses, with the aid of props, without strain or pain, we can achieve physical, mental and emotional relaxation. Restorative yoga classes are very relaxing and slow paced. Props, like blocks, bolsters, blankets and straps are used so that you are supported in your pose comfortably. You will then hold the pose for an extended period of time. This practice is great to balance an active yoga schedule or to give yourself a break when you feel under the weather.

Our parasympathetic nervous system is stimulated when we relax into poses, which promotes a relaxation response and reduces stress in our bodies. The parasympathetic nervous system is responsible for slowing your heart rate and breath and increasing blood flow to your vital organs, among other things.

When you are practicing restorative yoga, you will feel a sense of motionlessness and shapelessness, and this can lead you to feel some emotional discomfort and vulnerability. If this happens, stay with the breath and allow it to pass.

Benefits

Restorative yoga helps to combat the physical and mental effects of everyday stress, and eases common

ailments such as headaches, backaches, anxiety, and insomnia with the use of restful poses and deep breathing techniques.
• Deeply relaxes the body
• Stills the mind
• Improves capacity for healing and balancing
• Balances the nervous and immune system
• Boosts immunity

• **Enhances your mood**

Restorative Yoga for Self-Care
When was the last time that you took an hour for deep relaxation and rest? Restorative yoga is a practice of physical, emotional, and mental relaxation and rest. Practiced at a slow pace, restorative yoga focuses on stillness, holding gentle poses, and deep breathing. Restorative yoga can help to regulate the central nervous system and replenish your energy. It is so helpful to begin or maintain a consistent self-care practice, so we have more to give ourselves and others. This 60-minute restorative yoga class is just for you. This is an all levels class suitable for beginners and experienced yogis. You don't need to be flexible or fit.

Chapter no 9
Yoga Nitra for Restful Sleep

In the present speedy world, rest has turned into an extravagance as opposed to a need for some. The burdens of day to day existence, combined with the steady excitement from innovation, can unleash destruction on our capacity to accomplish relaxing rest. Yoga Nitra, frequently alluded to as "yogic rest," offers a strong answer for this cutting edge issue. In this thorough aide, we will investigate what Yoga Nitra is, its advantages, how to rehearse it, and ways to integrate it into your sleep time schedule.

What is Yoga Nitra?

Yoga Nitra is an efficient type of directed unwinding that prompts a condition of cognizant profound rest. It began from the old lessons of yoga and has been adjusted and refined throughout the years to suit present day ways of life. In contrast to customary rest, where the brain is oblivious, Yoga Nitra permits you to enter a condition of profound unwinding while at the same time remaining completely mindful and cognizant.

The Advantages of Yoga Nitra:

Advances Profound Unwinding: By efficiently loosening up the body and brain, Yoga Nitra initiates a condition of significant unwinding, considering profound revival.

Decreases Pressure and Nervousness: Through its quieting impact on the sensory system, Yoga Nidra reduces pressure and uneasiness, advancing a feeling of inward harmony and serenity.

Further develops Rest Quality:

Ordinary act of Yoga Nitra can essentially work on the nature of rest, making it more straightforward to nod off, stay unconscious, and wake up feeling revived.
Upgrades Mental Clearness and Concentration: Yoga Nitra helps clear the messiness of the brain, further developing fixation, center, and mental lucidity.

Supports Imagination and Instinct:

By getting to more profound layers of awareness, Yoga Nitra can animate imagination and instinct, opening secret possibilities inside.

Instructions to Practice Yoga Nitra:

Put things in place:

Find a peaceful and agreeable space where you will not be upset. Faint the lights, change the temperature as you would prefer, and accumulate any props like covers or cushions for added solace.

Expect an Agreeable Position:

Rests on your back in Svanasana (carcass present) with your arms by your sides, palms looking up, and legs somewhat separated. Cause any changes important to guarantee you to feel completely upheld and loose.

Follow a Directed Reflection:

You can either go to a Yoga Nitra class drove by a confirmed teacher or utilize a directed contemplation recording. The educator will lead you through a progression of unwinding methods, breath mindfulness, and perceptions to prompt a condition of profound unwinding.

Stay Mindful and Attentive:

All through the training, endeavor to keep a condition of loosened up mindfulness, noticing any sensations, contemplations, or feelings that emerge without connection or judgment.

Close Carefully:

At the point when the meeting is finished, continuously take your mindfulness back to your environmental elements, delicately squirm your fingers and toes, and gradually change back to a situated position. Pause for a minute to consider how you feel prior to continuing your day.

Ways to integrate Yoga Nitra into Your Sleep time Schedule:

Lay out a Predictable Practice:

Plan to rehearse Yoga Nitra consistently, in a perfect world before sleep time to set up your body and psyche for rest.

Limit Energizers:

Limit openness to electronic gadgets, caffeine, and animating exercises in the hours paving the way to sleep time to advance unwinding.

Make a Loosening up Sleep time Custom:

Integrate other quieting exercises like delicate extending, journaling, or tasting natural tea to indicate to your body that now is the ideal time to loosen up.

Try different things with Timing: Assuming that you find it trying to remain alert during Yoga Nitra practice, take a stab at exploring different avenues regarding various seasons of day to see what turns out best for you.

Be Patient and Diligent:

Like any new ability, dominating Yoga Nitra takes time and tolerance. Be predictable with your training and trust that the advantages will unfurl progressively after some time.

Conclusion:

In this present reality where rest is much of the time forfeited for efficiency, Yoga Nitra offers a powerful solution for accomplishing tranquil and reviving rest. By efficiently loosening up the body and brain, Yoga Nitra advances profound unwinding, diminishes pressure and uneasiness, further develops rest quality, improves mental lucidity and concentration, and lifts innovativeness and instinct. By integrating Yoga Nitra into your sleep time normal and following the tips framed in this aide, you can encounter the groundbreaking force of yogic rest and stir to a more dynamic and satisfying life.

Yoga indri, also known as yogic sleep, is an ancient practice intended to help your body relax while your mind is alert.

The goal is to achieve a state of consciousness between being awake and being asleep while guiding yourself through the four stages of brain wave activity. These stages are known as beta, alpha, theta, and delta.

Beta:

Beta waves are produced when your brain is actively engaged in mental activity, such as an active and engrossing conversation.

Alpha:

Alpha waves are slower, and indicate less arousal in the brain. These occur when your brain is resting after being in an aroused state, such as when you take a break after a long focus session.

Theta:

Theta waves also indicate less arousal in the brain, such as when you're zoning out or daydreaming.

Delta:

Delta waves have the slowest frequency, and occur while you are sleeping.

Benefits of Yoga Nitra

Proper use of yoga indri can help with your sleep onset, ensuring you fall asleep quickly and are able to stay asleep throughout the night. Other benefits of yoga indri include:

Helping calm your sympathetic nervous system, otherwise known as the "fight or flight" response, and fosters a feeling of soothing relaxation

Helping your body naturally release the sleep hormone melatonin and prepare your body to rest

Reducing anxiety and promoting serenity

Yoga indri has a long history of use supporting patients experiencing mental and physical conditions. It's been used to help patients with post-traumatic stress disorder (PTSD), anxiety, depression, and even diabetes and menstrual disorders.

One study found that both meditation and yoga indri was helpful in reducing anxiety, with yoga indri proving to have a more calming effect. [1]

Yoga indri is typically done via guided meditation with a yoga instructor, but you can also guide yourself through it. We'll talk more about this later.

What's the Difference Between Yoga Nitra and Other Yoga Practices?

Hatha Yoga is an umbrella term that includes many of the traditional forms of yoga practices in the United States. It's based on techniques that are meant to balance physical and mental health. This old system includes the use of breathing exercises and yoga postures known as asana.

Not all yoga includes movement or holding poses, in fact, Yoga indri literally means yogic sleep and doesn't include any movement at all.

While traditional yoga and yoga indri both center around the relation of mind to body, yoga indri dives further into the meditative aspect of the practice. Most forms of yoga put an emphasis on the asana, otherwise known as yoga poses.

Yoga indri however, is practiced solely from a position of total relaxation, known as the Corpse Pose. The Corpse Pose is simply lying flat on your back. This position can be practiced on the floor, in the comfort of your bed, or anywhere that allows you to completely relax your body.

Rather than using your body, yoga indri's purpose is based on mental exercise. The focus isn't on the physical poses, but on achieving a certain state of mind.

Can Yoga Nitra Help with Sleep Disorders?

It can! In fact, yoga indri could be an effective treatment option if you've been struggling with insomnia. While it can't resolve the issue, especially if you have chronic insomnia, it can be a very healthy and beneficial habit to get into to help yourself sleep.

Yoga Nitra For Insomnia

A study published by Sleep Science and Practice observed the effects that yoga nidra had on two insomnia patients— both older men with sleep problems. After their initial assessment, they were provided with five supervised yoga nidra sessions before practicing daily on their own for four weeks.

The researchers found that yoga indri can help treat chronic insomnia— especially when used to complement additional treatment options. [2]

Additionally, the participants experienced improved sleep quality after practicing yoga indri. They also saw improvements in depression and anxiety symptoms, as well as reduced stress levels.

Combining Traditional Yoga Poses with Yoga Nitra For Sleep Apnea

Yoga indri can help you relax before bed, supporting deeper and more restorative sleep. Combining it with more traditional yoga asana and movement can help you sleep better in some unexpected ways.

According to numerous studies, yoga poses and movement can be especially helpful for obstructive sleep apnea because of how it compliments CPAP therapy.

CPAP, or continuous positive airway pressure, uses a gentle, constant stream of pressurized air to open your airways and help you breathe normally as you sleep. It's the most effective and popular treatment for sleep apnea.

One study published by the Indian Journal of Otolaryngology and Head & Neck Surgery found that practicing yoga can be an effective complement to sleep apnea therapies like CPAP.

The study observed 37 patients with mild to severe OSA, or who complained of snoring. Each patient was assigned a series of yoga poses to practice over three months to help them with their nasal breathing, as well as to exercise the muscles in their faces and throats. [3]

Participants that adhered to their yoga practice saw a reduction in the severity of their OSA symptoms, as well as improvements in sleep quality, snoring frequency, and severity.

It's also worth noting that in this study, many of the participants were male, middle age, and overweight or obese.

Researchers also reported that most of the participants also saw a drop in their baseline body mass index (BMI) and neck circumference after 3 months. This is significant because excess body weight and neck circumference can obstruct your upper airway and contribute to your sleep apnea symptoms.

In short, the researchers found that a consistent yoga practice can help sleep apnea patients breathe and sleep better, especially when they followed their CPAP treatment.

So with all this in mind, you're probably wondering now:
"How do you practice yoga indri?"

It's a simple practice you can do from the comfort of your bedroom. Let's explore the practice so you can add it to your night routine to help improve your sleep.

How Do You Practice Yoga Nitra?

There are many yoga classes that offer yoga indri lessons, but you don't need an instructor. It's also an easy practice to do on your own once you know the process.

If you have a smartphone there are many apps, such as Yoga Nitra on the App Store or Google Play, as well as videos available online that can guide you through your yoga indri sleep meditation sessions. Here are a few things to do before you get started.

First, lie flat on your back in the Corpse Pose you can do this in bed, on a yoga mat, or on the Higher Dose PEMF mat. Make sure your head, spine, and lower back are relaxed and properly supported. You can use pillows or a yoga bolster to add more support if needed. Once comfortable, you can begin the mental process:

First, visualize a lifelong goal or something related to your health like better sleep or deep relaxation.
Set an intention for why you're practicing, and keep it in mind throughout the session.
Find a safe place in your mind. This helps you feel more at ease while you practice.
Be aware of your body. Focus on any sensations you feel this will help you reduce the tension there so you can relax.
Be aware of your breath. Notice how it enters and leaves your body, as well as how your abdomen rises

and falls as you breathe. This helps you slow down and breathe more deeply and evenly.

Acknowledge your feelings good or bad. When you process your feelings, you can help yourself work through them and feel more balanced.

Observe your thoughts as they happen. If any negative thoughts arise, think about more positive aspects of those thoughts. This helps prevent stress and tension while you're trying to enter that deep relaxation.

If you feel happy or joyful, embrace it!

Be aware of how you're feeling, and try observing those feelings outside of yourself. This can help you become more in tune with your feelings.

When you finish, spend a few minutes reflecting on your practice.

How do you feel? How can you bring the joy you felt into your daily life?

Use a sleep mask to block out any light or distractions that can take away from your practice.

Always practice somewhere quiet, and with minimal distractions.

Start with shorter sessions around 15 to 20 minutes. You can always move to longer sessions once you have more experience.

Your body cools down while you're at rest. Before you start, cover up with a blanket. This is especially important if you get cold easily.

Can't Sleep? Give Yoga Nitra a Try

Yoga is great for getting a good night's sleep thanks to its physical and emotional benefits. Yoga indri is an especially great way to help yourself get restful deep sleep. It can also reduce anxiety, and help you become more in touch with your emotions.

Yoga indri can also be helpful if you're suffering from occasional insomnia by reducing anxiety (often the cause of delayed sleep onset) and helping to provide calm and prepare your brain for sleep. As a whole, yoga can also complement CPAP therapy for sleep apnea by helping improve your breathing patterns and the muscle tone in your throat.

Still, struggling to fall asleep and get the restful sleep you need? We have many great resources available on our website including how to create a sleep environment to help you fall asleep more easily.

For more serious chronic insomnia conditions, our team of Advanced Practice Providers (APP) Sleep Specialists can diagnose and provide ongoing care for insomnia. They're trained in the most effective forms of treatment, including the first line of recommended treatment for insomnia. Contact us today for an evaluation. Our offices are located in Clarksville, Franklin, and Murfreesboro. We can help you get the attention you need to get a good night's sleep again.

Chapter no 10
Evening Reflection and Gratitude

In the buzzing about of present day life, it's not difficult to become involved with the hurricane of undertakings, commitments, and interruptions. In any case, setting aside some margin to stop and reflect at night can be unbelievably significant for our psychological, profound, and otherworldly prosperity. This act of night reflection and appreciation permits us to develop care, appreciate the gifts in our lives, and encourage a more profound feeling of satisfaction and satisfaction. In this intelligent article, we'll investigate the significance of night reflection, the advantages of developing appreciation, and down to earth procedures for coordinating these practices into our day to day routines.

The Significance of Night Reflection:

Evening reflection fills in as an extension between the exercises of the day and the relaxing time of rest. It gives a valuable chance to survey our encounters, contemplations, and feelings from the day with a feeling of interest and non-judgment. By carving out opportunity to reflect, we can acquire significant bits of knowledge into our ways of behaving, inspirations, and regions for development.

Reflection likewise permits us to commend our accomplishments, regardless of how little, and recognize the headway we've made towards our objectives. This feeling of achievement helps our confidence and persuades us to keep taking a stab at greatness in different parts of our lives.

Besides, evening reflection helps us loosen up and depressurize following a bustling day. It gives a space to unwinding and thoughtfulness, permitting us to deliver any repressed strain or stress gathered over the course of the day. By relinquishing stresses and nerves, we make mental space for quietness and inner harmony, which are fundamental for relaxing rest.

Advantages of Developing Appreciation:

Appreciation is the act of recognizing and valuing the beneficial things in our lives, regardless of how enormous or little. Research has shown that developing appreciation has various advantages for our psychological, profound, and actual wellbeing.

One of the essential advantages of appreciation is its positive effect on our state of mind and generally prosperity. At the point when we center around the gifts in our lives, we shift our consideration away from cynicism and shortage towards overflow and energy. This change in context can prompt expanded sensations of joy, fulfillment, and satisfaction.

Appreciation likewise encourages versatility notwithstanding misfortune. By perceiving the silver linings and illustrations in testing circumstances, we foster a more noteworthy feeling of internal strength and hopefulness. Rather than harping on mishaps or frustrations, we approach existence with an outlook of development and appreciation, which enables us to defeat snags and return more grounded than previously.

Besides, developing appreciation upgrades our connections and social associations. At the point when we express appreciation towards others, whether through words, signals, or thoughtful gestures, we reinforce the obligations of fellowship, love, and brotherhood. Appreciation encourages sympathy, empathy, and liberality, making a positive criticism circle of generosity and correspondence in our collaborations with others.

Down to earth Procedures for Night Reflection and Appreciation:

Now that we comprehend the significance and advantages of night reflection and appreciation, how about we investigate a few viable methodologies for incorporating these practices into our regular routines:

Keep an Appreciation Diary:

Distribute a couple of moments each night to record three things you're thankful for from the day. These can be basic delights, significant encounters, or thoughtful gestures from others. Considering these favors develops a feeling of appreciation and overflow in your life.

Practice Careful Contemplation:

Put away opportunity for a short care reflection before bed. Center around your breath and notice any considerations, feelings, or vibes that emerge without judgment. Careful reflection helps quiet the psyche, loosen up the body, and develop present second mindfulness, setting you up for soothing rest.

Consider Examples Learned:

Take a couple of seconds to ponder the illustrations and bits of knowledge **acquired** from the day's encounters, both positive and negative. Consider how you can apply these illustrations to future circumstances to develop and work on personally. Each experience, whether lovely or testing, offers a chance for development and learning.

Offer Thanks to Other people:

Regularly practice it to offer thanks to individuals in your day to day existence who emphatically affect you. Whether it's a sincere card to say thanks, a call, or a straightforward thoughtful gesture, let others in on the amount you value them and the commitments they make to your life.

Develop a Sleep time Schedule:

Make a relieving sleep time schedule that advances unwinding and readies your body and brain for rest. This could incorporate exercises like perusing a book, cleaning up, rehearsing delicate yoga, or paying attention to quieting music. Laying out a predictable sleep time routine signs to your body that now is the ideal time to slow down and change into relaxing rest.

Conclusion:

Evening reflection and appreciation are strong practices that support the spirit, develop care, and improve our general prosperity. By finding opportunity to consider our encounters, offer thanks for our favors, and develop a feeling of inward harmony and happiness, we make an establishment for living a more significant and satisfying life. As we coordinate these practices into our day to day routines, may we embrace each night as a chance for self-revelation, development, and appreciation.

Your natural state is inner happiness and satisfaction. In this state you feel vital, healthy, and alive, less influenced by negative thoughts and emotions.

However, you won't fully enjoy this state if your physical, emotional, mental and subtle (spiritual) dimensions are out of alignment.

For example, if your physical body is out of alignment, you might experience chronic health conditions like joint pain, fatigue or difficulty maintaining a healthy weight.

Emotionally you may experience overwhelm, sadness, anger or frustration. You may choose to numb your pain with alcohol, drugs or overeating.

Mentally you may notice difficulty concentrating, or being caught up in a pattern of negative thoughts that shift your focus to a negative place perpetuating the cycle.

You may even be out of touch with what brings you real joy and fulfillment in life.

Recognitions, featuring High-Tech Meditation and The Holistic Lifestyle, is a powerful tool to help you realign yourself and enjoy your natural state on a consistent basis.

With High-Tech Meditation you can more quickly:

1. Enjoy a natural high as the release of endorphins associated with meditation allows you to relax and de-stress from daily challenges.

2. Enjoy the elevated well-being associated with whole-brain functioning like improved decision making and enhanced ability to concentrate.

3. Build a bridge between the logical, analytical capabilities of your brain's left hemisphere and the imaginative, intuitive ones of the right, expanding creativity, flow and productivity.

4. Achieve greater objectivity and perspective that can help you maintain calm in all situations.

5. Tap into deeper states of consciousness where you will enjoy inner stillness, harmony and balance in your physical, emotional and mental dimensions.

7. Reduce your unconscious reactions to people and events that trigger an emotional response; reactions that trap you in past anger or future anxiety and keep you from enjoying the present moment.

8. Expand your emotional clearing process and release energy for more enjoyable pursuits.

9. Enjoy higher levels of wellness as reduced stress levels promote healthier bodies, emotions and minds.

10. Increase self-love, acceptance, and happiness.